The Definitive Medite
Recipe Gu

Quick and Easy Recipes to Amazingl
Get Back in Shape

Ava Foster

Table of contents

Honey Almond–Crusted Chicken Tenders

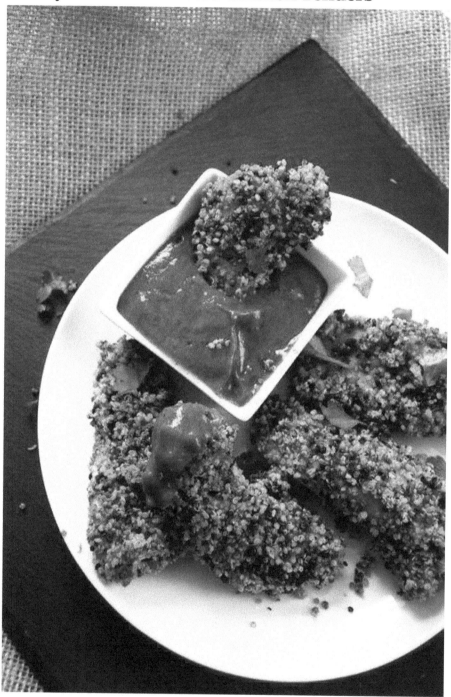

Difficulty Level: 3/5

Preparation time: 10 *minutes*

Cooking time: 10 *minutes*

Servings: 4

Ingredients:

Nonstick cooking spray

1 tablespoon honey

1 tablespoon whole-grain or Dijon mustard

¼ teaspoon kosher or sea salt

¼ teaspoon freshly ground black pepper

1 pound boneless, skinless chicken breast tenders or tenderloins

1 cup almonds (about 3 ounces)

Directions:

Preheat the oven to 425°F. Line a large, rimmed baking sheet with parchment paper. Place a wire cooling rack on the parchment-lined baking sheet, and coat the rack well with nonstick cooking spray.

In a large bowl, combine the honey, mustard, salt, and pepper. Add the chicken and stir gently to coat. Set aside.

Use a knife or a mini food processor to chop the almonds roughly; they should be about the size of sunflower seeds. Dump the nuts onto a large sheet of parchment paper and spread them out. Press the coated chicken tenders into the nuts until evenly coated on all sides. Place the chicken on the prepared wire rack.

Bake for 15 to 20 minutes, or until the internal temperature of the chicken measures 165°F on a meat thermometer and any juices run clear. Serve immediately.

Nutrition:

Per serving

Calories: 263

Total fat: 12g

Saturated fat: 1g

Cholesterol: 65mg

Sodium: 237mg

Potassium: 85mg

Total Carbohydrates: 9g

Fiber: 3g

Protein: 31g

Romesco Poached Chicken

Difficulty Level: 2/5

Preparation time: 5 *minutes*

Cooking time: 20 *minutes*

Servings: 6

Ingredients:

1½ pounds boneless, skinless chicken breasts, cut into 6 pieces

1 carrot, halved

1 celery stalk, halved

½ onion, halved

2 garlic cloves, smashed

3 sprigs fresh thyme or rosemary

1 cup Romesco Dip

2 tablespoons chopped fresh flat-leaf (Italian) parsley

¼ teaspoon freshly ground black pepper

Directions:

Put the chicken in a medium saucepan. Fill with water until there's about one inch of liquid above the chicken. Add the carrot, celery, onion, garlic, and thyme. Cover and bring it to a boil. Reduce the heat to low (keeping it covered), and cook for 12 to 15 minutes, or until the internal temperature of the chicken measures 165°F on a meat thermometer and any juices run clear.

Remove the chicken from the water and let sit for 5 minutes.

When you're ready to serve, spread ¾ cup of romesco dip on the bottom of a serving platter. Arrange the chicken breasts on top, and drizzle with the remaining romesco dip. Sprinkle the tops with parsley and pepper.

Nutrition:

Per serving

Calories: 237

Total fat: 11g

Saturated fat: 1g

Cholesterol: 65mg

Total Carbohydrates: 8g

Fiber: 4g

Protein: 28g

Roasted Red Pepper Chicken with Lemony Garlic Hummus

Difficulty Level: 2/5

Preparation time: 10 *minutes*

Cooking time: 10 *minutes*

Servings: 6

Ingredients:

1¼ pounds boneless, skinless chicken thighs, cut into 1-inch pieces

½ sweet or red onion, cut into 1-inch chunks (about 1 cup)

2 tablespoons extra-virgin olive oil

½ teaspoon dried thyme

¼ teaspoon freshly ground black pepper

¼ teaspoon kosher or sea salt

1 (12-ounce) jar roasted red peppers, drained and chopped

Lemony Garlic Hummus, or a 10-ounce container prepared hummus

½ medium lemon

3 (6-inch) whole-wheat pita breads, cut into eighths

Directions:

Line a large, rimmed baking sheet with aluminum foil. Set aside. Set one oven rack about 4 inches below the broiler element. Preheat the broiler to high.

In a large bowl, mix together the chicken, onion, oil, thyme, pepper, and salt. Spread the mixture onto the prepared baking sheet.

Place the chicken under the broiler and broil for 5 minutes. Remove the pan, stir in the red peppers, and return to the broiler. Broil for another

5 minutes, or until the chicken and onion just start to char on the tips. Remove from the oven.

Spread the hummus onto a large serving platter, and spoon the chicken mixture on top. Squeeze the juice from half a lemon over the top, and serve with the pita pieces.

Nutrition:

Per serving

Calories: 324

Total fat: 11g

Saturated fat: 2g

Cholesterol: 54mg

Sodium: 625mg

Total Carbohydrates: 29g

Fiber: 6g

Protein: 29g

Sheet Pan Lemon Chicken and Roasted Artichokes

Difficulty Level: 3/5

Preparation time: 10 *minutes*

Cooking time: *20 minutes*

Servings: *4*

Ingredients:

2 large lemons

3 tablespoons extra-virgin olive oil, divided

½ teaspoon kosher or sea salt

2 large artichokes

4 (6-ounce) bone-in, skin-on chicken thighs

Directions:

Put a large, rimmed baking sheet in the oven. Preheat the oven to 450°F with the pan inside. Tear off four sheets of aluminum foil about 8-by-10 inches each; set aside.

Using a Microplane or citrus zester, zest 1 lemon into a large bowl. Halve both lemons and squeeze all the juice into the bowl with the zest. Whisk in 2 tablespoons of oil and the salt. Set aside.

Rinse the artichokes with cool water, and dry with a clean towel. Using a sharp knife, cut about 1½ inches off the tip of each artichoke. Cut about ¼ inch off each stem. Halve each artichoke lengthwise so each piece has equal amounts of stem. Immediately plunge the artichoke halves into the lemon juice and oil mixture (to prevent browning) and turn to coat on all sides. Lay one artichoke half flat-side down in the center of a sheet of aluminum foil, and close up loosely to make a foil packet. Repeat the process with the remaining three artichoke halves. Set the packets aside.

Put the chicken in the remaining lemon juice mixture and turn to coat.

Using oven mitts, carefully remove the hot baking sheet from the oven and pour on the remaining tablespoon of oil; tilt the pan to coat. Carefully arrange the chicken, skin-side down, on the hot baking sheet. Place the artichoke packets, flat-side down, on the baking sheet as well. (Arrange the artichoke packets and chicken with space between them so air can circulate around them.)

Roast for 20 minutes, or until the internal temperature of the chicken measures 165°F on a meat thermometer and any juices run clear. Before serving, check the artichokes for doneness by pulling on a leaf. If it comes out easily, the artichoke is ready.

Nutrition:

Per serving

Calories: 372

Total fat: 11g

Saturated fat: 29g

Cholesterol: 98mg

Sodium: 381mg

Total Carbohydrates: 11g

Fiber: 5g

Protein: 20g

Roasted Tomato Pita Pizzas

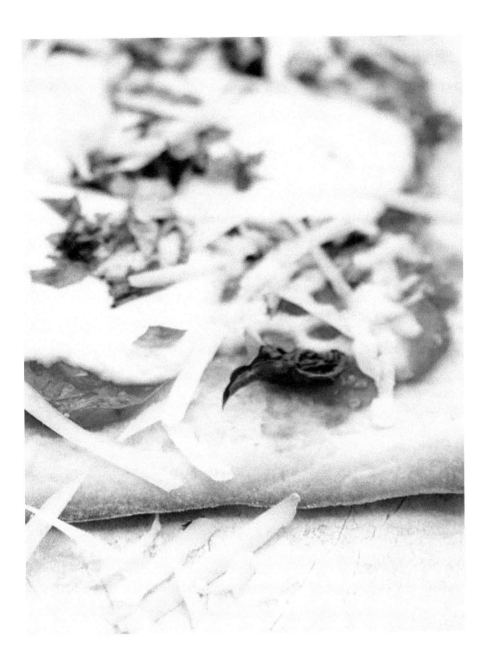

Difficulty Level: 3/5

Preparation time: 10 *minutes*

Cooking time: 20 *minutes*

Servings: 6

Ingredients:

2 pints grape tomatoes (about 3 cups), halved

1 tablespoon extra-virgin olive oil

2 garlic cloves, minced (about 1 teaspoon)

1 teaspoon chopped fresh thyme leaves (from about 6 sprigs)

¼ teaspoon freshly ground black pepper

¼ teaspoon kosher or sea salt

¾ cup shredded Parmesan cheese (about 3 ounces)

6 whole-wheat pita breads

Directions:

Preheat the oven to 425°F.

In a baking pan, mix together the tomatoes, oil, garlic, thyme, pepper, and salt. Roast for 10 minutes. Pull out the rack, stir the tomatoes with a spatula or wooden spoon while still in the oven, and mash down the softened tomatoes to release more of their liquid. Roast for an additional 10 minutes.

While the tomatoes are roasting, sprinkle 2 tablespoons of cheese over each pita bread. Place the pitas on a large, rimmed baking sheet and toast in the oven for the last 5 minutes of the tomato cooking time.

Remove the tomato sauce and pita bread from the oven. Stir the tomatoes, spoon about ⅓ cup of sauce over each pita bread, and serve.

Nutrition:

Per serving

Calories: 259

Total fat: 7g

Saturated fat: 3g

Cholesterol: 10mg

Sodium: 555mg

Total Carbohydrates: 40g

Fiber: 6g

Protein: 12g

No-Drain Pasta alla Norma

Difficulty Level: 3/5

Preparation time: 5 *minutes*

Cooking time: 15 *minutes*

Servings: 6

Ingredients:

1 medium globe eggplant (about 1 pound), cut into ¾-inch cubes

1 tablespoon extra-virgin olive oil

1 cup chopped onion (about ½ medium onion)

8 ounces uncooked thin spaghetti

1 (15-ounce) container part-skim ricotta cheese

3 Roma tomatoes, chopped (about 2 cups)

2 garlic cloves, minced (about 1 teaspoon)

¼ teaspoon kosher or sea salt

½ cup loosely packed fresh basil leaves

Grated Parmesan cheese, for serving (optional)

Directions:

Lay three paper towels on a large plate, and pile the cubed eggplant on top. (Don't cover the eggplant.) Microwave the eggplant on high for 5 minutes to dry and partially cook it.

In a large stockpot over medium-high heat, heat the oil. Add the eggplant and the onion and cook for 5 minutes, stirring occasionally.

Add the spaghetti, ricotta, tomatoes, garlic, and salt. Cover with water by a ½ inch (about 4 cups of water). Cook uncovered for 12 to 15 minutes, or until the pasta is just al dente (tender with a bite), stirring

18

occasionally to prevent the pasta from sticking together or sticking to the bottom of the pot.

Remove the pot from the heat and let the pasta stand for 3 more minutes to absorb more liquid while you tear the basil into pieces. Sprinkle the basil over the pasta and gently stir. Serve with Parmesan cheese, if desired.

Prep tip: We use the microwave in this recipe to partially cook and moisten the eggplant, making it less spongy and less likely to sop up oil. We use a similar moistening trick in the Israeli Eggplant, Chickpea, and Mint Sauté by broiling the eggplant to make it silky smooth.

Nutrition:

Per serving

Calories: 389

Total fat: 9g

Saturated fat: 4g

Cholesterol: 22mg

Sodium: 177mg

Total Carbohydrates: 62g

Fiber: 4g

Protein: 19g

Zucchini with Bow Ties

Difficulty Level: 2/5

Preparation time: 5 *minutes*

Cooking time: 15 *minutes*

Servings: *4*

Ingredients:

3 tablespoons extra-virgin olive oil

2 garlic cloves, minced (about 1 teaspoon)

3 large or 4 medium zucchini, diced (about 4 cups)

½ teaspoon freshly ground black pepper

¼ teaspoon kosher or sea salt

½ cup 2% milk

¼ teaspoon ground nutmeg

8 ounces uncooked farfalle (bow ties) or other small pasta shape

½ cup grated Parmesan or Romano cheese (about 2 ounces)

1 tablespoon freshly squeezed lemon juice (from ½ medium lemon)

Directions:

In a large skillet over medium heat, heat the oil. Add the garlic and cook for 1 minute, stirring frequently. Add the zucchini, pepper, and salt. Stir well, cover, and cook for 15 minutes, stirring once or twice.

In a small, microwave-safe bowl, warm the milk in the microwave on high for 30 seconds. Stir the milk and nutmeg into the skillet and cook uncovered for another 5 minutes, stirring occasionally.

While the zucchini is cooking, in a large stockpot, cook the pasta according to the package directions.

Drain the pasta in a colander, saving about 2 tablespoons of pasta water. Add the pasta and pasta water to the skillet. Mix everything together and remove from the heat. Stir in the cheese and lemon juice and serve.

Nutrition:

Per serving

Calories: 410

Total fat: 17g

Saturated fat: 4g

Cholesterol: 13mg

Sodium: 382mg

Total Carbohydrates: 45g

Fiber: 4g

Protein: 15g

Roasted Asparagus Caprese Pasta

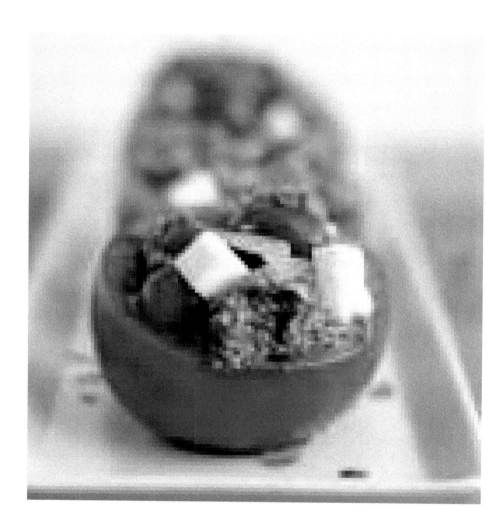

Difficulty Level: 2/5

Preparation time: 10 *minutes*

Cooking time: 15 *minutes*

Servings: 6

Ingredients:

8 ounces uncooked small pasta, like orecchiette (little ears) or farfalle (bow ties)

1½ pounds fresh asparagus, ends trimmed and stalks chopped into 1-inch pieces (about 3 cups)

1 pint grape tomatoes, halved (about 1½ cups)

2 tablespoons extra-virgin olive oil

¼ teaspoon freshly ground black pepper

¼ teaspoon kosher or sea salt

2 cups fresh mozzarella, drained and cut into bite-size pieces (about 8 ounces)

⅓ cup torn fresh basil leaves

2 tablespoons balsamic vinegar

Directions:

Preheat the oven to 400°F.

In a large stockpot, cook the pasta according to the package directions. Drain, reserving about ¼ cup of the pasta water.

While the pasta is cooking, in a large bowl, toss the asparagus, tomatoes, oil, pepper, and salt together. Spread the mixture onto a large, rimmed baking sheet and bake for 15 minutes, stirring twice as it cooks.

Remove the vegetables from the oven, and add the cooked pasta to the baking sheet. Mix with a few tablespoons of pasta water to help the sauce become smoother and the saucy vegetables stick to the pasta.

Gently mix in the mozzarella and basil. Drizzle with the balsamic vinegar. Serve from the baking sheet or pour the pasta into a large bowl.

If you want to make this dish ahead of time or to serve it cold, follow the recipe up to step 4, then refrigerate the pasta and vegetables. When you are ready to serve, follow step 5 either with the cold pasta or with warm pasta that's been gently reheated in a pot on the stove.

Nutrition:

Per serving

Calories: 307

Total fat: 14g

Saturated fat: 6g

Cholesterol: 29mg

Sodium: 318mg

Total Carbohydrates: 33g

Fiber: 9g

Protein: 18g

Speedy Tilapia with Red Onion and Avocado

Difficulty Level: 2/5

Preparation time: 10 *minutes*

Cooking time: 5 *minutes*

Servings: *4*

Ingredients:

1 tablespoon extra-virgin olive oil

1 tablespoon freshly squeezed orange juice

¼ teaspoon kosher or sea salt

4 (4-ounce) tilapia fillets, more oblong than square, skin-on or skinned

¼ cup chopped red onion (about ⅛ onion)

1 avocado, pitted, skinned, and sliced

Directions:

In a 9-inch glass pie dish, use a fork to mix together the oil, orange juice, and salt. Working with one fillet at a time, place each in the pie dish and turn to coat on all sides. Arrange the fillets in a wagon-wheel formation, so that one end of each fillet is in the center of the dish and the other end is temporarily draped over the edge of the dish. Top each fillet with 1 tablespoon of onion, then fold the end of the fillet that's hanging over the edge in half over the onion. When finished, you should have 4 folded-over fillets with the fold against the outer edge of the dish and the ends all in the center.

Cover the dish with plastic wrap, leaving a small part open at the edge to vent the steam. Microwave on high for about 3 minutes. The fish is done when it just begins to separate into flakes (chunks) when pressed gently with a fork.

Top the fillets with the avocado and serve.

Prep tip: Because most fish skin is relatively thin, it cooks at about the same rate as fish flesh, which is why you can use this microwave method for both skin-on and skinless fish.

Nutrition:

Per serving

Calories: 200

Total fat: 11g

Saturated fat: 2g

Cholesterol: 55mg

Sodium: 161mg

Total Carbohydrates: 4g

Fiber: 3g

Protein: 22g

Grilled Fish on Lemons

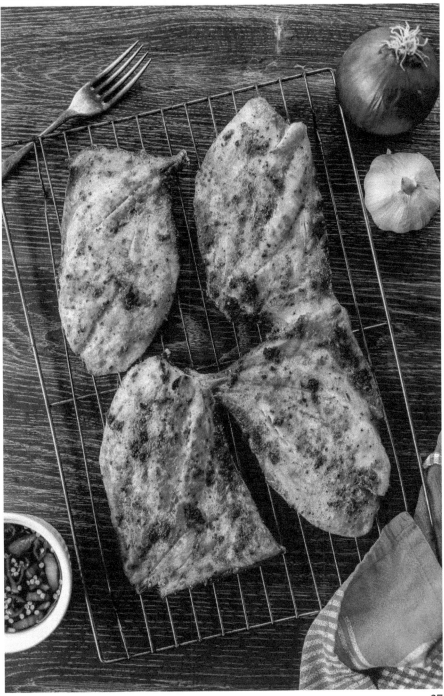

Difficulty Level: 3/5

Preparation time: 10 *minutes*

Cooking time: 10 *minutes*

Servings: *4*

Ingredients:

4 (4-ounce) fish fillets, such as tilapia, salmon, catfish, cod, or your favorite fish

Nonstick cooking spray

3 to 4 medium lemons

1 tablespoon extra-virgin olive oil

¼ teaspoon freshly ground black pepper

¼ teaspoon kosher or sea salt

Directions:

Using paper towels, pat the fillets dry and let stand at room temperature for 10 minutes. Meanwhile, coat the cold cooking grate of the grill with nonstick cooking spray, and preheat the grill to 400°F, or medium-high heat. Or preheat a grill pan over medium-high heat on the stove top.

Cut one lemon in half and set half aside. Slice the remaining half of that lemon and the remaining lemons into ¼-inch-thick slices. (You should have about 12 to 16 lemon slices.) Into a small bowl, squeeze 1 tablespoon of juice out of the reserved lemon half.

Add the oil to the bowl with the lemon juice, and mix well. Brush both sides of the fish with the oil mixture, and sprinkle evenly with pepper and salt.

Carefully place the lemon slices on the grill (or the grill pan), arranging 3 to 4 slices together in the shape of a fish fillet, and repeat with the remaining slices. Place the fish fillets directly on top of the lemon slices, and grill with the lid closed. (If you're grilling on the stove top, cover with a large pot lid or aluminum foil.) Turn the fish halfway through the cooking time only if the fillets are more than half an inch thick. (See tip for cooking time.) The fish is done and ready to serve when it just begins to separate into flakes (chunks) when pressed gently with a fork.

Nutrition:

Per serving

Calories: 147

Total fat: 5g

Saturated fat: 1g

Cholesterol: 55mg

Sodium: 158mg

Total Carbohydrates: 4g

Fiber: 1g

Protein: 22g

Weeknight Sheet Pan Fish Dinner

Difficulty Level: 2/5

Preparation time: 10 *minutes*

Cooking time: 10 *minutes*

Servings: *4*

Ingredients:

Nonstick cooking spray

2 tablespoons extra-virgin olive oil

1 tablespoon balsamic vinegar

4 (4-ounce) fish fillets, such as cod or tilapia (½ inch thick)

2½ cups green beans (about 12 ounces)

1 pint cherry or grape tomatoes (about 2 cups

Directions:

Preheat the oven to 400°F. Coat two large, rimmed baking sheets with nonstick cooking spray.

In a small bowl, whisk together the oil and vinegar. Set aside.

Place two pieces of fish on each baking sheet.

In a large bowl, combine the beans and tomatoes. Pour in the oil and vinegar, and toss gently to coat. Pour half of the green bean mixture over the fish on one baking sheet, and the remaining half over the fish on the other. Turn the fish over, and rub it in the oil mixture to coat. Spread the vegetables evenly on the baking sheets so hot air can circulate around them.

Bake for 5 to 8 minutes, until the fish is just opaque and not translucent. The fish is done and ready to serve when it just begins to separate into flakes (chunks) when pressed gently with a fork.

Nutrition:

Per serving

Calories: 193

Total fat: 8g

Saturated fat: 2g

Cholesterol: 55mg

Sodium: 49mg

Total Carbohydrates: 8g

Fiber: 3g

Protein: 23g

Crispy Polenta Fish Sticks
Difficulty Level: 2/5

Preparation time: 15 minutes

Cooking time: 10 minutes

Servings: 4

Ingredients:

2 large eggs, lightly beaten 1 tablespoon 2% milk

1 pound skinned fish fillets (cod, tilapia, or other white fish) about ½ inch thick, sliced into 20 (1-inch-wide) strips

½ cup yellow cornmeal

½ cup whole-wheat panko bread crumbs or whole-wheat bread crumbs

¼ teaspoon smoked paprika

¼ teaspoon kosher or sea salt

¼ teaspoon freshly ground black pepper

Nonstick cooking spray

Directions:

Place a large, rimmed baking sheet in the oven. Preheat the oven to 400°F with the pan inside.

In a large bowl, mix the eggs and milk. Using a fork, add the fish strips to the egg mixture and stir gently to coat.

Put the cornmeal, bread crumbs, smoked paprika, salt, and pepper in a quart-size zip-top plastic bag. Using a fork or tongs, transfer the fish to the bag, letting the excess egg wash drip off into the bowl before transferring. Seal the bag and shake gently to coat each fish stick completely.

With oven mitts, carefully remove the hot baking sheet from the oven and spray it with nonstick cooking spray. Using a fork or tongs, remove the fish sticks from the bag and arrange them on the hot baking sheet, with space between them so the hot air can circulate and crisp them up.

Bake for 5 to 8 minutes, until gentle pressure with a fork causes the fish to flake, and serve.

Nutrition:

Per serving

Calories: 256

Total fat: 6g

Saturated fat: 1g

Cholesterol: 148mg

Sodium: 321mg

Total Carbohydrates: 22g

Fiber: 2g

Protein: 29g

Salmon Skillet Supper
Difficulty Level: 2/5

Preparation time: 5 minutes

Cooking time: 15 minutes

Servings: 4

Ingredients:

1 tablespoon extra-virgin olive oil

2 garlic cloves, minced (about 1 teaspoon)

1 teaspoon smoked paprika

1 pint grape or cherry tomatoes, quartered (about 1½ cups)

1 (12-ounce) jar roasted red peppers, drained and chopped

1 tablespoon water

¼ teaspoon freshly ground black pepper

¼ teaspoon kosher or sea salt

1 pound salmon fillets, skin removed, cut into 8 pieces

1 tablespoon freshly squeezed lemon juice (from ½ medium lemon)

Directions:

In a large skillet over medium heat, heat the oil. Add the garlic and smoked paprika and cook for 1 minute, stirring often. Add the tomatoes, roasted peppers, water, black pepper, and salt. Turn up the heat to medium-high, bring to a simmer, and cook for 3 minutes, stirring occasionally and smashing the tomatoes with a wooden spoon toward the end of the cooking time.

Add the salmon to the skillet, and spoon some of the sauce over the top. Cover and cook for 10 to 12 minutes, or until the salmon is cooked through (145°F using a meat thermometer) and just starts to flake.

Remove the skillet from the heat, and drizzle lemon juice over the top of the fish. Stir the sauce, then break up the salmon into chunks with a fork. You can serve it straight from the skillet.

Nutrition:

Per serving

Calories: 289

Total fat: 13g

Saturated fat: 2g

Cholesterol: 68mg

Sodium: 393mg

Total Carbohydrates: 10g

Fiber: 2g

Protein: 31g

Orange and Garlic Shrimp
Difficulty Level: 2/5

Preparation time: 20 minutes

Cooking time: 10 minutes

Servings: 6

Ingredients:

1 large orange

3 tablespoons extra-virgin olive oil, divided

1 tablespoon chopped fresh rosemary (about 3 sprigs) or 1 teaspoon dried rosemary

1 tablespoon chopped fresh thyme (about 6 sprigs) or 1 teaspoon dried thyme

3 garlic cloves, minced (about 1½ teaspoons)

¼ teaspoon freshly ground black pepper

¼ teaspoon kosher or sea salt

1½ pounds fresh raw shrimp, (or frozen and thawed raw shrimp) shells and tails removed

Directions:

Zest the entire orange using a Microplane or citrus grater.

In a large zip-top plastic bag, combine the orange zest and 2 tablespoons of oil with the rosemary, thyme, garlic, pepper, and salt. Add the shrimp, seal the bag, and gently massage the shrimp until all the ingredients are combined and the shrimp is completely covered with the seasonings. Set aside.

Heat a grill, grill pan, or a large skillet over medium heat. Brush on or swirl in the remaining 1 tablespoon of oil. Add half the shrimp, and cook for 4 to 6 minutes, or until the shrimp turn pink and white, flipping halfway through if on the grill or stirring every minute if in a pan. Transfer the shrimp to a large serving bowl. Repeat with the remaining shrimp, and add them to the bowl.

While the shrimp cook, peel the orange and cut the flesh into bite-size pieces. Add to the serving bowl, and toss with the cooked shrimp. Serve immediately or refrigerate and serve cold.

Nutrition:

Per serving

Calories: 190

Total fat: 8g

Saturated fat: 1g

Cholesterol: 221mg

Sodium: 215mg

Total Carbohydrates: 4g

Fiber: 1g

Protein: 24g

Greek Stuffed Collard Greens

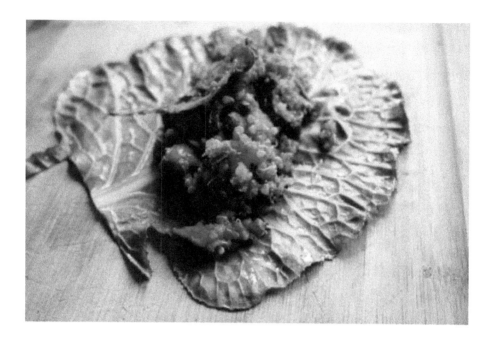

Difficulty Level: 3/5

Preparation time: 10 minutes

Cooking time: 20 minutes

Servings: 4

Ingredients:

1 (28-ounce) can low-sodium or no-salt-added crushed tomatoes

8 collard green leaves (about ⅓ pound), tough tips of stems cut off

1 recipe Mediterranean Lentils and Rice or 2 (10-ounce) bags frozen grain medley (about 4 cups), cooked

2 tablespoons grated Parmesan cheese

Directions:

Preheat the oven to 400°F. Pour the tomatoes into a baking pan and set aside.

Fill a large stockpot about three-quarters of the way with water and bring to a boil. Add the collard greens and cook for 2 minutes. Drain in a colander. Put the greens on a clean towel or paper towels and blot dry.

To assemble the stuffed collards, lay one leaf flat on the counter vertically. Add about ½ cup of the lentils and rice mixture to the middle of the leaf, and spread it evenly along the middle of the leaf. Fold one long side of the leaf over the rice filling, then fold over the other long side so it is slightly overlapping. Take the bottom end, where the stem was, and gently but firmly roll up until you have a slightly square package. Carefully transfer the stuffed leaf to the baking pan, and place it seam-side down in the crushed tomatoes. Repeat with the remaining leaves.

Sprinkle the leaves with the grated cheese, and cover the pan with aluminum foil. Bake for 20 minutes, or until the collards are tender-firm, and serve. (If you prefer softer greens, bake for an additional 10 minutes.)

Nutrition:

Per serving

Calories: 205

Total fat: 8g

Saturated fat: 2g

Cholesterol: 3mg

Sodium: 524mg

Total Carbohydrates: 34g

Fiber: 8g

Protein: 6g

Powerhouse Arugula Salad
Difficulty Level: 1/5

Preparation time: 10 minutes

Cooking time: 0 minutes

Servings: 4

Ingredients:

4 tablespoons extra-virgin olive oil

Zest and juice of 2 clementines or 1 orange (2 to 3 tablespoons)

1 tablespoon red wine vinegar

½ teaspoon sålt

¼ teaspoon freshly ground black pepper

8 cups baby arugula

1 cup coarsely chopped walnuts

1 cup crumbled goat cheese

½ cup pomegranate seeds

Directions:

In a small bowl, whisk together the olive oil, zest and juice, vinegar, salt, and pepper and set aside.

To assemble the salad for serving, in a large bowl, combine the arugula, walnuts, goat cheese, and pomegranate seeds. Drizzle with the dressing and toss to coat.

Nutrition:

Per serving

Calories: 444

Total fat: 40g

Sodium: 412mg

Total Carbohydrates: 11g

Fiber: 3g

Protein: 10g

Avocado Gazpacho

Difficulty Level: 1/5

Preparation time: 15 minutes

Cooking time: 0 minutes

Servings: 4

Ingredients:

2 cups chopped tomatoes

2 large ripe avocados, halved and pitted

1 large cucumber, peeled and seeded

1 medium bell pepper (red, orange or yellow), chopped

1 cup plain whole-milk Greek yogurt

¼ cup extra-virgin olive oil

¼ cup chopped fresh cilantro

¼ cup chopped scallions, green part only

2 tablespoons red wine vinegar

Juice of 2 limes or 1 lemon

½ to 1 teaspoon salt

¼ teaspoon freshly ground black pepper

Directions:

In a blender or in a large bowl, if using an immersion blender, combine the tomatoes, avocados, cucumber, bell pepper, yogurt, olive oil, cilantro, scallions, vinegar, and lime juice. Blend until smooth. If using a stand blender, you may need to blend in two or three batches.

Season with salt and pepper and blend to combine the flavors.

Chill in the refrigerator for 1 to 2 hours before serving. Serve cold.

Nutrition:

Per serving

Calories: 392

Total fat: 32g

Sodium: 335mg

Total Carbohydrates: 20g

Fiber: 9g

Protein: 6g

Dilled Tuna Salad Sandwich

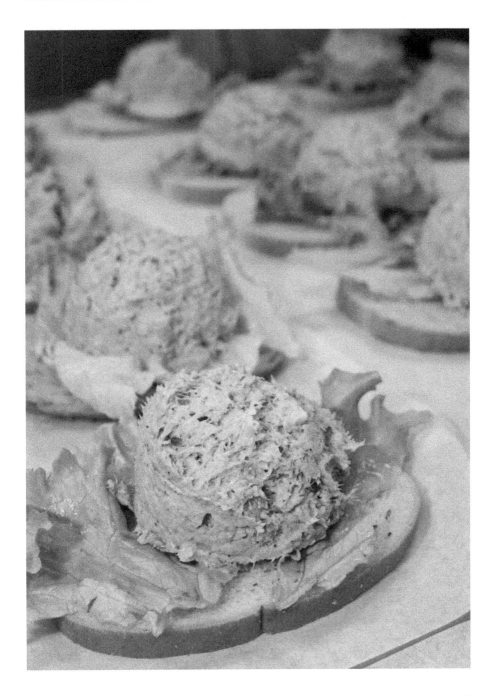

Difficulty Level: 1/5

Preparation time: 10 minutes

Cooking time: 0 minutes

Servings: 4

Ingredients:

4 Versatile Sandwich Rounds

2 (4-ounce) cans tuna, packed in olive oil

2 tablespoons Roasted Garlic Aioli, or avocado oil mayonnaise with 1 to 2 teaspoons freshly squeezed lemon juice and/or zest

1 very ripe avocado, peeled, pitted, and mashed

1 tablespoon chopped fresh capers (optional)

1 teaspoon chopped fresh dill or ½ teaspoon dried dill

Directions:

Make sandwich rounds according to recipe. Cut each round in half and set aside.

In a medium bowl, place the tuna and the oil from cans. Add the aioli, avocado, capers (if using), and dill and blend well with a fork.

Toast sandwich rounds and fill each with one-quarter of the tuna salad, about ⅓ cup.

Nutrition:

Per serving (1 sandwich)

Calories: 436

Total fat: 36g

Sodium: 790mg

Total Carbohydrates: 5g

Fiber: 3g

Protein: 23g

Orange-Tarragon Chicken Salad Wrap

Difficulty Level: 1/5

Preparation time: 15 minutes

Cooking time: 0 minutes

Servings: 4

Ingredients:

½ cup plain whole-milk Greek yogurt

2 tablespoons Dijon mustard

2 tablespoons extra-virgin olive oil

2 tablespoons chopped fresh tarragon or 1 teaspoon dried tarragon

½ teaspoon salt

¼ teaspoon freshly ground black pepper

2 cups cooked shredded chicken

½ cup slivered almonds

4 to 8 large Bibb lettuce leaves, tough stem removed

2 small ripe avocados, peeled and thinly sliced

Zest of 1 clementine, or ½ small orange (about 1 tablespoon)

Directions:

In a medium bowl, combine the yogurt, mustard, olive oil, tarragon, orange zest, salt, and pepper and whisk until creamy.

Add the shredded chicken and almonds and stir to coat.

To assemble the wraps, place about ½ cup chicken salad mixture in the center of each lettuce leaf and top with sliced avocados.

Nutrition:

Per serving

Calories: 440

Total fat: 32g

Sodium: 445mg

Total Carbohydrates: 12g

Fiber: 8g

Protein: 26g

Versatile Sandwich Round
Difficulty Level: 1/5

Preparation time: 5 minutes

Cooking time: 90 seconds

Servings: 1

Ingredients:

3 tablespoons almond flour

1 tablespoon extra-virgin olive oil

1 large egg

½ teaspoon dried rosemary, oregano, basil, thyme, or garlic powder (optional)

¼ teaspoon baking powder

⅛ teaspoon salt

Directions:

In a microwave-safe ramekin, combine the almond flour, olive oil, egg, rosemary (if using), baking powder, and salt. Mix well with a fork.

Microwave for 90 seconds on high.

Slide a knife around the edges of ramekin and flip to remove the bread.

Slice in half with a serrated knife if you want to use it to make a sandwich.

Nutrition:

Per serving

Calories: 232

Total fat: 22g

Sodium: 450mg

Total Carbohydrates: 1g

Fiber: 0g

Protein: 8g

Caprese Grilled Cheese

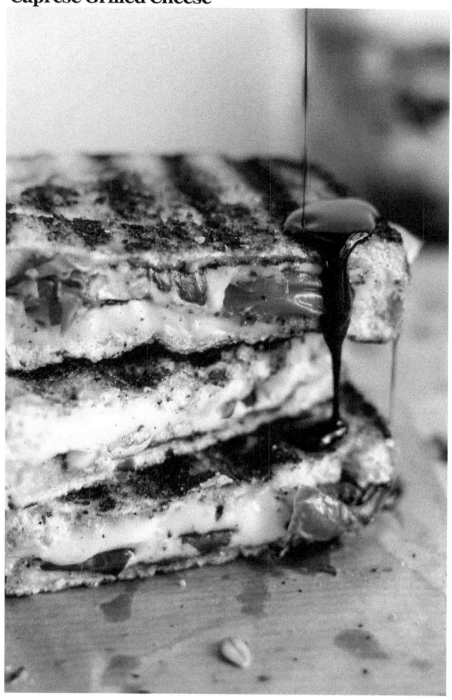

Difficulty Level: 2/5

Preparation time: 10 minutes

Cooking time: 10 minutes

Servings: 4

Ingredients:

4 <u>Versatile Sandwich Rounds</u>

8 tablespoons jarred pesto

4 ounces fresh mozzarella cheese, cut into 4 round slices

1 Roma tomato or small slicing tomato, cut into 4 slices

4 tablespoons extra-virgin olive oil

Directions:

In a microwave-safe ramekin, combine the almond flour, olive oil, egg, rosemary (if using), baking powder, and salt. Mix well with a fork.

Microwave for 90 seconds on high.

Slide a knife around the edges of ramekin and flip to remove the bread.

Slice in half with a serrated knife if you want to use it to make a sandwich.

Nutrition:

Per serving

Calories: 232

Total fat: 22g

Sodium: 450mg

Total Carbohydrates: 1g

Fiber: 0g

Protein: 8g

Riced Cauliflower

Difficulty Level: 2/5

Preparation time: 5 minutes

Cooking time: 10 minutes

Servings: 6-8

Ingredients:

1 small head cauliflower, broken into florets

¼ cup extra-virgin olive oil

2 garlic cloves, finely minced

1½ teaspoons salt

½ teaspoon freshly ground black pepper

Directions:

Place the florets in a food processor and pulse several times, until the cauliflower is the consistency of rice or couscous.

In a large skillet, heat the olive oil over medium-high heat. Add the cauliflower, garlic, salt, and pepper and sauté for 5 minutes, just to take the crunch out but not enough to let the cauliflower become soggy.

Remove the cauliflower from the skillet and place in a bowl until ready to use. Toss with chopped herbs and additional olive oil for a simple side, top with sautéed veggies and protein, or use in your favorite recipe.

Nutrition:

Per serving

Calories: 92

Total fat: 9g

Sodium: 595mg

Total Carbohydrates: 3g

Fiber: 1g

Protein: 1g

Greek Chicken and "Rice" Soup with Artichokes

Difficulty Level: 2/5

Preparation time: 10 minutes

Cooking time: 15 minutes

Servings: 4

Ingredients:

4 cups chicken stock

2 cups <u>Riced Cauliflower</u>, divided

2 large egg yolks

¼ cup freshly squeezed lemon juice (about 2 lemons)

¾ cup extra-virgin olive oil, divided

8 ounces cooked chicken, coarsely chopped

1 (13.75-ounce) can artichoke hearts, drained and quartered

¼ cup chopped fresh dill

Directions:

In a large saucepan, bring the stock to a low boil. Reduce the heat to low and simmer, covered.

Transfer 1 cup of the hot stock to a blender or food processor. Add ½ cup raw riced cauliflower, the egg yolks, and lemon juice and purée. While the processor or blender is running, stream in ½ cup olive oil and blend until smooth.

Whisking constantly, pour the purée into the simmering stock until well blended together and smooth. Add the chicken and artichokes and simmer until thickened slightly, 8 to 10 minutes. Stir in the dill and remaining 1½ cups riced cauliflower. Serve warm, drizzled with the remaining ¼ cup olive oil.

Nutrition:

Per serving

Calories: 566

Total fat: 46g

Sodium: 754mg

Total Carbohydrates: 14g

Fiber: 7g

Protein: 24g

Citrus Asparagus with Pistachios
Difficulty Level: 2/5

Preparation time: 10 minutes

Cooking time: 15 minutes

Servings: 4

Ingredients:

5 tablespoons extra-virgin olive oil, divided

Zest and juice of 2 clementines or 1 orange (about ¼ cup juice and 1 tablespoon zest)

Zest and juice of 1 lemon

1 tablespoon red wine vinegar

1 teaspoon salt, divided

¼ teaspoon freshly ground black pepper

½ cup shelled pistachios

1 pound fresh asparagus

1 tablespoon water

Directions:

In a small bowl, whisk together 4 tablespoons olive oil, the clementine and lemon juices and zests, vinegar, ½ teaspoon salt, and pepper. Set aside.

In a medium dry skillet, toast the pistachios over medium-high heat until lightly browned, 2 to 3 minutes, being careful not to let them burn. Transfer to a cutting board and coarsely chop. Set aside.

Trim the rough ends off the asparagus, usually the last 1 to 2 inches of each spear. In a skillet, heat the remaining 1 tablespoon olive oil over medium-high heat. Add the asparagus and sauté for 2 to 3 minutes. Sprinkle with the remaining ½ teaspoon salt and add the water. Reduce the heat to medium-low, cover, and cook until tender, another 2 to 4 minutes, depending on the thickness of the spears.

Transfer the cooked asparagus to a serving dish. Add the pistachios to the dressing and whisk to combine. Pour the dressing over the warm asparagus and toss to coat.

Nutrition:

Per serving

Calories: 284

Total fat: 24g

Sodium: 594mg

Total Carbohydrates: 11g

Fiber: 4g

Protein: 6g

Garlicky Shrimp with Mushrooms

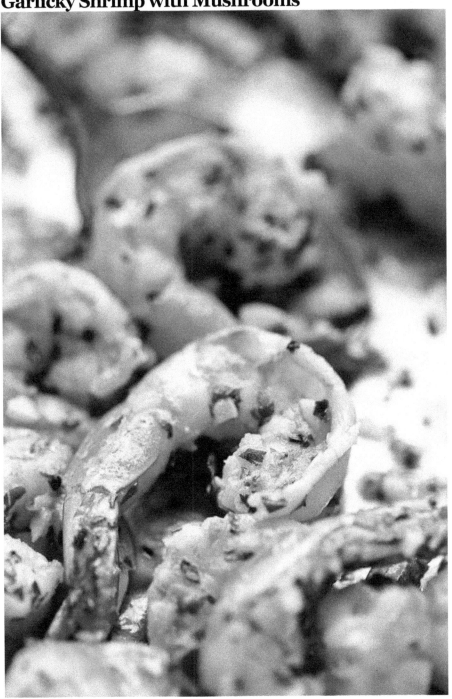

Difficulty Level: 2/5

Preparation time: 10 minutes

Cooking time: 15 minutes

Servings: 4

Ingredients:

1 pound peeled and deveined fresh shrimp

1 teaspoon salt

1 cup extra-virgin olive oil

8 large garlic cloves, thinly sliced

4 ounces sliced mushrooms (shiitake, baby bella, or button)

½ teaspoon red pepper flakes

¼ cup chopped fresh flat-leaf Italian parsley

Zucchini Noodles or Riced Cauliflower, for serving

Directions:

In a small bowl, whisk together 4 tablespoons olive oil, the clementine and lemon juices and zests, vinegar, ½ teaspoon salt, and pepper. Set aside.

In a medium dry skillet, toast the pistachios over medium-high heat until lightly browned, 2 to 3 minutes, being careful not to let them burn. Transfer to a cutting board and coarsely chop. Set aside.

Trim the rough ends off the asparagus, usually the last 1 to 2 inches of each spear. In a skillet, heat the remaining 1 tablespoon olive oil over medium-high heat. Add the asparagus and sauté for 2 to 3 minutes. Sprinkle with the remaining ½ teaspoon salt and add the water. Reduce the heat to medium-low, cover, and cook until tender, another 2 to 4 minutes, depending on the thickness of the spears.

Transfer the cooked asparagus to a serving dish. Add the pistachios to the dressing and whisk to combine. Pour the dressing over the warm asparagus and toss to coat.

Nutrition:

Per serving

Calories: 284

Total fat: 24g

Sodium: 594mg

Total Carbohydrates: 11g

Fiber: 4g

Protein: 6g

Zucchini Noodles
Difficulty Level: 1/5

Preparation time: 5 minutes

Cooking time: 0 minutes

Servings: 4

Ingredients:

2 medium to large zucchini

Directions:

Cut off and discard the ends of each zucchini and, using a spiralizer set to the smallest setting, spiralize the zucchini to create zoodles.

To serve, simply place a ½ cup or so of spiralized zucchini into the bottom of each bowl and spoon a hot sauce over top to "cook" the zoodles to al dente consistency. Use with any of your favorite sauces, or just toss with warmed pesto for a simple and quick meal.

Nutrition:

Per serving

Calories: 48

Total fat: 1g

Sodium: 7mg

Total Carbohydrates: 7g

Fiber: 3g

Protein: 6g

Cod with Parsley Pistou
Difficulty Level: 2/5

Preparation time: 15 minutes

Cooking time: 10 minutes

Servings: 4

Ingredients:

1 cup packed roughly chopped fresh flat-leaf Italian parsley

1 to 2 small garlic cloves, minced

Zest and juice of 1 lemon

1 teaspoon salt

½ teaspoon freshly ground black pepper

1 cup extra-virgin olive oil, divided

1 pound cod fillets, cut into 4 equal-sized pieces

Directions:

In a food processer, combine the parsley, garlic, lemon zest and juice, salt, and pepper. Pulse to chop well.

While the food processor is running, slowly stream in ¾ cup olive oil until well combined. Set aside.

In a large skillet, heat the remaining ¼ cup olive oil over medium-high heat. Add the cod fillets, cover, and cook 4 to 5 minutes on each side, or until cooked through. Thicker fillets may require a bit more cooking time. Remove from the heat and keep warm.

Add the pistou to the skillet and heat over medium-low heat. Return the cooked fish to the skillet, flipping to coat in the sauce. Serve warm, covered with pistou.

Nutrition:

Calories: 581

Total Fat: 55g,

Total Carbohydrates: 3g,

Net Carbohydrates: 2g,

Fiber: 1g,

Protein: 21g;

Sodium: 652mg

Rosemary-Lemon Snapper Baked in Parchment
Difficulty Level: 2/5

Preparation time: 15 minutes

Cooking time: 15 minutes

Servings: 4

Ingredients:

1¼ pounds fresh red snapper fillet, cut into two equal pieces

2 lemons, thinly sliced

6 to 8 sprigs fresh rosemary, stems removed or 1 to 2 tablespoons dried rosemary

½ cup extra-virgin olive oil

6 garlic cloves, thinly sliced

1 teaspoon salt

½ teaspoon freshly ground black pepper

Directions:

Preheat the oven to 425°F.

Place two large sheets of parchment (about twice the size of each piece of fish) on the counter. Place 1 piece of fish in the center of each sheet.

Top the fish pieces with lemon slices and rosemary leaves.

In a small bowl, combine the olive oil, garlic, salt, and pepper. Drizzle the oil over each piece of fish.

5 . Top each piece of fish with a second large sheet of parchment and starting on a long side, fold the paper up to about 1 inch from the fish. Repeat on the remaining sides, going in a clockwise direction. Fold in each corner once to secure.

Place both parchment pouches on a baking sheet and bake until the fish is cooked through, 10 to 12 minutes.

Nutrition:

Calories: 390,

Total Fat: 29g,

Total Carbohydrates: 3g,

Net Carbohydrates: 3g,

Fiber: 0g,

Protein: 29g;

Sodium: 674mg

Shrimp in Creamy Pesto over Zoodles

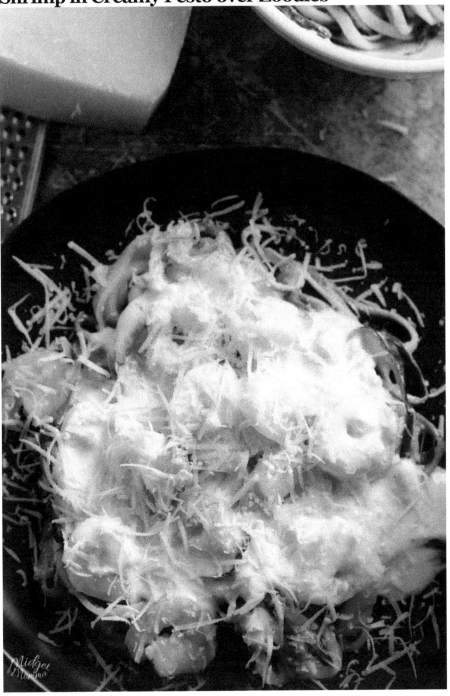

Difficulty Level: 2/5

Preparation time: 10 minutes

Cooking time: 10 minutes

Servings: 4

Ingredients:

1 pound peeled and deveined fresh shrimp

Salt

Freshly ground black pepper

2 tablespoons extra-virgin olive oil

½ small onion, slivered

8 ounces store-bought jarred pesto

¾ cup crumbled goat or feta cheese, plus more for serving

6 cups Zucchini Noodles (from about 2 large zucchini), for serving

¼ cup chopped flat-leaf Italian parsley, for garnish

Directions:

In a bowl, season the shrimp with salt and pepper and set aside.

In a large skillet, heat the olive oil over medium-high heat. Sauté the onion until just golden, 5 to 6 minutes.

Reduce the heat to low and add the pesto and cheese, whisking to combine and melt the cheese. Bring to a low simmer and add the shrimp. Reduce the heat back to low and cover. Cook until the shrimp is cooked through and pink, another 3 to 4 minutes.

Serve warm over Zucchini Noodles, garnishing with chopped parsley and additional crumbled cheese, if desired.

Nutrition:

Calories: 491,

Total Fat: 35g,

Total Carbohydrates: 15g,

Net Carbohydrates: 11g,

Fiber: 4g,

Protein: 29g;

Sodium: 870mg

Nut-Crusted Baked Fish

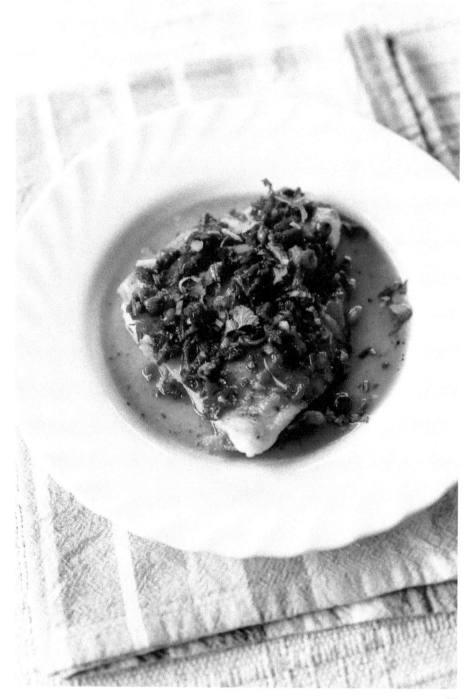

Difficulty Level: 2/5

Preparation time: 10 minutes

Cooking time: 20 minutes

Servings: 4

Ingredients:

½ cup extra-virgin olive oil, divided

1 pound flaky white fish (such as cod, haddock, or halibut), skin removed

½ cup shelled finely chopped pistachios

½ cup ground flaxseed

Zest and juice of 1 lemon, divided

1 teaspoon ground cumin

1 teaspoon ground allspice

½ teaspoon salt (use 1 teaspoon if pistachios are unsalted)

¼ teaspoon freshly ground black pepper

Directions:

Preheat the oven to 400°F.

Line a baking sheet with parchment paper or aluminum foil and drizzle 2 tablespoons olive oil over the sheet, spreading to coat the bottom evenly.

Cut the fish into 4 equal pieces and place on the prepared baking sheet.

In a small bowl, combine the pistachios, flaxseed, lemon zest, cumin, allspice, salt, and pepper. Drizzle in ¼ cup olive oil and stir well.

Divide the nut mixture evenly atop the fish pieces. Drizzle the lemon juice and remaining 2 tablespoons oil over the fish and bake until cooked through, 15 to 20 minutes, depending on the thickness of the fish.

Nutrition:

Calories: 509,

Total Fat: 41g,

Total Carbohydrates: 9g,

Net Carbohydrates: 3g,

Fiber: 6g,

Protein: 26g;

Sodium: 331mg

Pesto Walnut Noodles
Difficulty Level: 2/5

Preparation time: 10 minutes

Cooking time: 15 minutes

Servings: 4

Ingredients:

4 Zucchini, Made into Zoodles

¼ Cup Olive Oil, Divided

½ Teaspoon Crushed Red Pepper

2 Cloves Garlic, Minced & Divided

¼ Teaspoon Black Pepper

¼ Teaspoon sea Salt

2 Tablespoons Parmesan Cheese, Grated & Divided

1 Cup Basil, Fresh & Packed

¾ Cup Walnut Pieces, Divided

Directions:

Start by making your zucchini noodles by using a spiralizer to get ribbons. Combine your zoodles with a minced garlic clove and tablespoon of oil. Season with salt and pepper and crushed red pepper. Set it to the side.

Get out a large skillet and heat a ½ a tablespoon of oil over medium-high heat. Add in half of your zoodles, cooking for five minutes. You will need to stir every minute or so. Repeat with another ½ a tablespoon of oil and your remaining zoodles.

Make your pesto while your zoodles cook. Put your garlic clove, a tablespoon or parmesan, basil leaves and ¼ cup of walnuts in your food processor. Season with salt and pepper if desired, and drizzle the remaining two tablespoons of oil in until completely blended.

Add the pesto to your zoodles, topping with remaining walnuts and parmesan to serve.

Nutrition:

Calories: 301

Protein: 7 Grams

Fat: 28 Grams

Carbohydrates: 11 Grams

Sodium: 160 mg

Tomato Tabbouleh

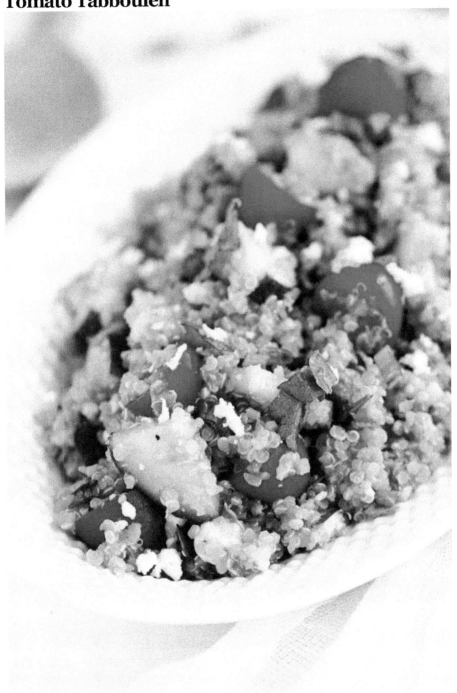

Difficulty Level: 2/5

Preparation time: 10 minutes

Cooking time: 20 minutes

Servings: 4

Ingredients:

8 Beefsteak Tomatoes

½ Cup Water

3 Tablespoons Olive Oil, Divided

½ Cup Whole Wheat Couscous, Uncooked

1 ½ Cups Parsley, Fresh & Minced

2 Scallions Chopped

1/3 Cup Mint, Fresh & Minced

Sea Salt & Black Pepper to Taste

1 Lemon

4 Teaspoons Honey, Raw

1/3 Cup Almonds, Chopped

Directions:

Start by heating your oven to 400 degrees. Take your tomato and slice the top off each one before scooping the flesh out. Put the tops flesh and seeds in a mixing bowl.

Get out a baking dish before adding in a tablespoon of oil to grease it. Place your tomatoes in the dish, and then cover your dish with foil.

Now you will make your couscous while your tomatoes cook. Bring the water to a boil using a saucepan and then add the couscous in and cover. Remove it from heat, and allow it to sit for five minutes. Fluff it with a fork.

Chop your tomato flesh and tops up, and then drain the excess water using a colander. Measure a cup of your chopped tomatoes and place them back in the mixing bowl. Mix with mint scallions, pepper, salt and parsley.

Zest your lemon into the bowl, and then half the lemon. Squeeze the lemon juice in, and mix well.

Add your tomato mix to the couscous.

Carefully remove your tomatoes from the oven and then divide your tabbouleh among your tomatoes. Cover the pan with foil and then put it in the oven. Cook for another eight to ten minutes. Your tomatoes should be firm but still tender.

Drizzle with honey and top with almonds before serving.

Nutrition:
Calories: 314

Protein: 8 Grams

Fat: 15 Grams

Carbohydrates: 41 Grams

Sodium: 141

Lemon Faro Bowl
Difficulty Level: 2/5

Preparation time: 10 minutes

Cooking time: 15 minutes

Servings: 6

Ingredients:

1 Tablespoon + 2 Teaspoons Olive Oil, Divided

1 Cup Onion, Chopped

2 Cloves Garlic, Minced

1 Carrot, Shredded

2 Cups Vegetable Broth, Low Sodium

1 Cup Pearled Faro

2 Avocados, Peeled, Pitted & Sliced

1 Lemon, Small

Sea Salt to Taste

Directions:

Start by placing a saucepan over medium-high heat. Add in a tablespoon of oil and then throw in your onion once the oil is hot. Cook for about five minutes, stirring frequently to keep it from burning.

Add in your carrot and garlic. Allow it to cook for about another minute while you continue to stir.

Add in your broth and faro. Allow it to come to a boil and adjust your heat to high to help. Once it boils, lower it to medium-low and cover your saucepan. Let it simmer for twenty minutes. The faro should be al dente and plump.

Pour the faro into a bowl and add in your avocado and zest. Drizzle with your remaining oil and add in your lemon wedges.

Nutrition:
Calories: 279

Protein: 7 Grams

Fat: 14 Grams

Carbohydrates: 36 Grams

Sodium: 118 mg

Chickpea & Red Pepper Delight

Difficulty Level: 2/5

Preparation time: 15 minutes

Cooking time: 15 minutes

Servings: 3

Ingredients:

1 Red Bell Pepper, Diced

2 Cups Water

4 Sun-Dried Tomatoes

¼ Cup Red Wine Vinegar

2 Tablespoon Olive Oil

2 Cloves Garlic, Chopped

29 Ounces Chickpeas, Canned, Drained & Rinsed

½ Cup Parsley, Chopped / Sea Salt to Taste

Directions:

Get a baking sheet and put your red bell pepper on it with the skin side up.

Bake for eight minutes. Your skin should bubble, and then place it in a bag to seal it.

Remove your bell peppers in about ten minutes, and then slice it into thin slices.

Get out two cups of water and pour it in a bowl. Microwave for four minutes and add in your sundried tomatoes, letting them sit for ten minutes. Drain them before slicing into thin strips. Mix your red wine vinegar and garlic with your olive oil. Ross your roasted red bell pepper with parsley, sun dried tomatoes, and chickpeas. Season with salt before serving.

Nutrition:

Calories: 195

Protein: 9.3 Grams

Fat: 8.5 Grams

Carbohydrates: 25.5 Grams

Sodium: 142 mg

Chickpea Salad
Difficulty Level: 2/5

Preparation time: 10 minutes

Cooking time: 0 minutes

Servings: 6

Ingredients:

28 ounces chickpeas, drained

½ red onion, chopped fine

2 cucumbers, chopped fine

¼ cup olive oil

2 lemons, juiced

1 lemon, zested

1 tablespoon tahini

3 cloves garlic, minced

2 teaspoons oregano

Sea salt & black pepper to taste

Directions:

Get a bowl and combine your cucumbers with your chickpeas and red onion.

Get a small bowl and whisk your lemon juice, olive oil, lemon zest, tahini, garlic, sea salt, oregano and pepper.

Toss the dressing with your salad before serving.

Nutrition:
Calories: 231

Protein: 12 Grams

Fat: 12 Grams

Carbohydrates: 8 Grams

Sodium: 160 mg

Eggplant Rolls

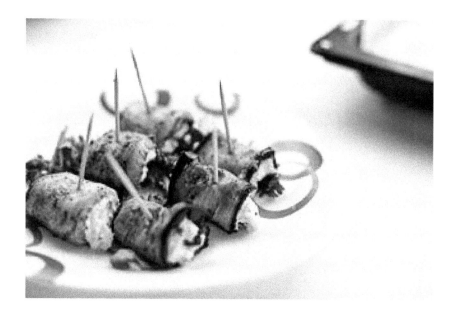

Difficulty Level: 2/5

 Preparation time: 10 minutes

Cooking time: 6 minutes

Servings: 6

Ingredients:

1 eggplant, ½ inch sliced lengthwise

Sea salt & black pepper to taste

1 tablespoon olive oil

1/3 cup cream cheese

½ cup tomatoes, chopped

1 clove garlic, minced

2 tablespoons dill, chopped

Directions:

Slice your eggplant before brushing it down with olive oil. Season your eggplant slices with salt and pepper.

Grill the eggplants for three minutes per side.

Get out a bowl and combine cream cheese, garlic, dill and tomatoes in a different bowl.

Allow your eggplant slices to cool and then spread the mixture over each one. Roll them and pin them with a toothpick to serve.

Nutrition:
Calories: 91

Protein: 2.1 Grams

Fat: 7 Grams

Carbohydrates: 6.3 Grams

Sodium: 140 mg

Heavenly Quinoa
Difficulty Level: 2/5

Preparation time: 15 minutes

Cooking time: 5 minutes

Servings: 5

Ingredients:

1 cup almonds

1 cup quinoa

1 teaspoon cinnamon

1 pinch sea salt

1 teaspoon vanilla extract, pure

2 cups milk

2 tablespoons honey, raw

3 dates, dried, pitted & chopped fine

5 apricots, dried & chopped fine

Directions:

Get out a skillet to toast your almonds in for about five minutes. They should be golden and aromatic.

Place your quinoa and cinnamon in a saucepan using medium heat. Add in your vanilla, salt and milk. Stir and then bring it to a boil. Reduce your heat, and allow it to simmer for fifteen minutes.

Add in your dates, honey, apricots and half of your almonds.

Serve topped with almonds and parsley if desired.

Nutrition:
Calories: 344

Protein: 12.6 Grams

Fat: 13.8 Grams

Carbohydrates: 45.7 Grams

Sodium: 96 mg

Red Bean & Green Salad
Difficulty Level: 2/5

Preparation time: 10 minutes

Cooking time: 0 minutes

Servings: 6

Ingredients:

1 cup red beans, cooked & drained

1 cup lettuce, shredded & chopped

2 cups spinach leaves

1 cup red onions, sliced into thin rings

½ cup walnuts, halved

3 tablespoon olive oil

3 tablespoons lemon juice, fresh

1 clove garlic, minced

1 teaspoon dijon mustard

¼ teaspoon sea salt, fine / ¼ teaspoon black pepper

Directions:

Combine your lettuce, spinach, walnut, red beans and red onion together.

In a different bowl mix your olive oil, garlic, Dijon mustard and lemon juice together to form your dressing.

Drizzle the dressing over the salad and adjust salt and pepper as necessary.

Serve immediately.

Nutrition:
Calories: 242

Protein: 10.1 Grams

Fat: 13.7 Grams

Carbohydrates: 22.7 Grams

Sodium: 121 mg

Chickpea Patties

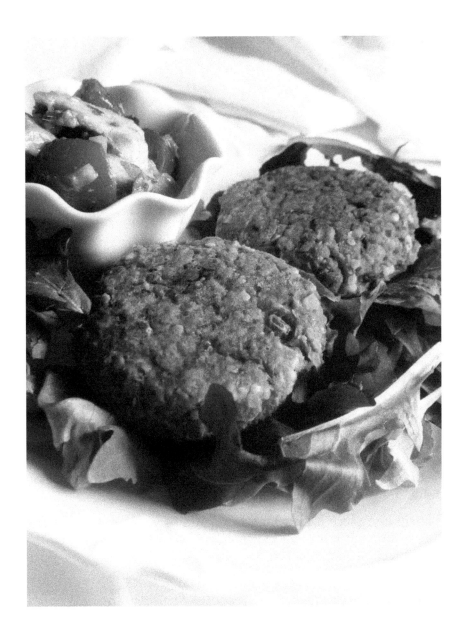

Difficulty Level: 2/5

Preparation time: 10 minutes

Cooking time: 15 minutes

Servings: 8

Ingredients:

1 Cup Flour

¾ Cup hot water

1 egg, whisked

½ teaspoon cumin

½ teaspoon sea salt, fine

1 cup spinach, fresh & chopped

3 cloves garlic, minced

1/8 teaspoon baking soda

¾ cup chickpeas, cooked

2 scallions, small & chopped

1 cup olive oil

Directions:

Get a bowl and mix your salt, cumin and flour together. Add in your water and egg to form a batter. Whisk well. It should thicken.

Stir in your baking soda, garlic, spinach, chickpeas, and scallions, blending well.

Get a pan and place it over high heat. Add in your oil. Once your oil begins to simmer, pour in a tablespoon of your batter, frying on both sides. Repeat until all your batter is used.

Garnish with lime and greens before serving.

Nutrition:
Calories: 352

Protein: 6.1 Grams

Fat: 27.1 Grams

Carbohydrates: 24 Grams

Sodium: 160 mg

Red Onion Tilapia
Difficulty Level: 2/5

Preparation time: 10 minutes

Cooking time: 5 minutes

Servings: 4

Ingredients:

1 tablespoon olive oil

1 tablespoon orange juice, fresh

¼ teaspoon sea salt, fine

1 avocado, pitted, skinned & sliced

¼ cup red onion, chopped

4 tilapia fillets, 4 ounces each

Directions:

Start by getting out a pie dish that is nine inches. Glass is best. Use a fork to mix your slat, orange juice and oil together. Dip one filet at a time and then put them in your dish. They should be coated on both sides. Put them in a wheel formation so that each fillet is in the center of the dish and draped over the edge. Top each fillet with a tablespoon of onion. Fold the fillet that's hanging over your pie dish in half so that it's over the onion.

Cover it with plastic wrap but don't close it all the way. They should be able to vent the steam. Microwave for three minutes.

Tip with avocado to serve.

Nutrition:
Calories: 200

Protein: 22 Grams

Fat: 11 Grams

Carbohydrates: 4 Grams

Sodium: 151

Chicken & Asparagus
Difficulty Level: 2/5

Preparation time: 10 minutes

Cooking time: 10 minutes

Servings: 4

Ingredients:

1 lb. Chicken breast, boneless & skinless

¼ cup flour

4 tablespoons butter

½ teaspoon sea salt, fine

½ teaspoon black pepper

1 teaspoon lemon pepper seasoning

2 slices lemon

1-2 cups asparagus, chopped

2 tablespoons honey, raw

Parsley to garnish

Directions:

Cover your chicken using plastic wrap and beat it until it's ¾ of an inch thick.

Get out a bowl and mix your slat, flour and pepper together. Coat your chicken in your flour mixture.

Get out a pan to melt two tablespoons of butter over medium-high heat.

Place the chicken breast in the pan to cook for three to five minutes. It should turn golden brown on each side.

While your chicken is cooking sprinkle the lemon on each side. Once it's cooked, transfer it to a plate. In the same pan add in your asparagus, cooking until it's crisp but tender. It should turn a bright green. Set it to the side.

You'll use the same pan to add your lemon slices to caramelize.

Nutrition:
Calories: 530

Protein: 36.8 Grams

Fat: 33.3 Grams

Carbohydrates: 28.8 Grams

Sodium: 130 mg

Beef Kofta

Difficulty Level: 2/5

Preparation time: 15 minutes

Cooking time: 15 minutes

Servings: 4

Ingredients:

1 lb. Ground beef, 93% lean or more

½ cup onions, minced

1 tablespoon olive oil

½ teaspoon sea salt, fine

½ teaspoon coriander, ground

½ teaspoon cumin, ground

¼ teaspoon cinnamon

¼ teaspoon mint leaves, dried

¼ teaspoon allspice

Directions:

Mix your beef, salt, cumin, coriander, cinnamon, oil, onion, mint and allspice together in a large bowl.

Get out wooden skewers and shape beef kebabs from the mixture.

Refrigerate for ten minutes before grilling them. You will need to preheat your grill and cook them for fourteen minutes. Remember to turn them constantly to avoid burning.

Serve warm.

Nutrition:
Calories: 216

Protein: 26.1 Grams

Fat: 12.2 Grams

Carbohydrates: 1.3 Grams

Sodium: 152 mg

Raisin Rice Pilaf

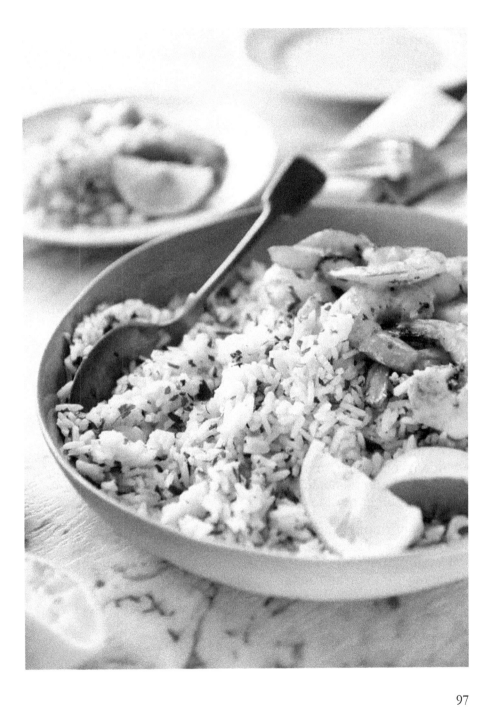

Difficulty Level: 2/5

Preparation time: 5 minutes

Cooking time: 15 minutes

Servings: 4

Ingredients:

1 tablespoon olive oil

1 teaspoon cumin

1 cup onion, chopped

½ cup carrot, shredded

½ teaspoon cinnamon

2 cups instant brown rice

1 ¾ cup orange juice

1 cup golden raisins

¼ cup water

½ cup pistachios, shelled

Fresh Chives, Chopped for Garnish

Directions:

Place a medium saucepan over medium-high heat before adding in your oil. Add n your onion, and stir often so it doesn't burn. Cook for about five minutes and then add in your cumin, cinnamon and carrot. Cook for about another minute.

Add in your orange juice, water and rice. Bring it all to a boil before covering your saucepan. Turn the heat down to medium-low and then allow it to simmer for six to seven minutes. Your rice should be cooked all the way through, and all the liquid should be absorbed.

Stir in your pistachios, chives and raisins. Serve warm.

Nutrition:
Calories: 320

Protein: 6 Grams

Fat: 7 Grams

Carbohydrates: 61 Grams

Sodium: 37 mg

Lebanese Delight

Difficulty Level: 2/5

Preparation time: 5 minutes

Cooking time: 25 minutes

Servings: 5

Ingredients:

1 tablespoon olive oil

1 cup vermicelli (can be substituted for thin spaghetti) broken into 1 to 1 ½ inch pieces

3 cups cabbage, shredded

3 cups vegetable broth, low sodium

½ cup water

1 cup instant brown rice

¼ teaspoon sea salt, fine

2 cloves garlic

¼ teaspoon crushed red pepper

½ cup cilantro fresh & chopped

Lemon slices to garnish

Directions:

Get a saucepan and then place it over medium-high heat. Add in your oil and once it's hot you will need to add in your pasta. Cook for three minutes or until your pasta is toasted. You will have to stir often in order to keep it from burning.

Add in your cabbage, cooking for another four minutes. Continue to stir often.

Add in your water and rice. Season with salt, red pepper and garlic before bringing it all to a boil over high heat. Stir, and then cover. Once it's covered turn the heat down to medium-low. Allow it all to simmer for ten minutes.

Remove the pan from the burner and then allow it to sit without lifting the lid for five minutes. Take the garlic cloves out and then mash them using a fork. Place them back in, and stir them into the rice. Stir in your cilantro as well and serve warm. Garnish with lemon wedges if desired.

Nutrition:
Calories: 259

Protein: 7 Grams

Fat: 4 Grams

Carbohydrates: 49 Grams

Sodium: 123 mg

Flavorful Braised Kale

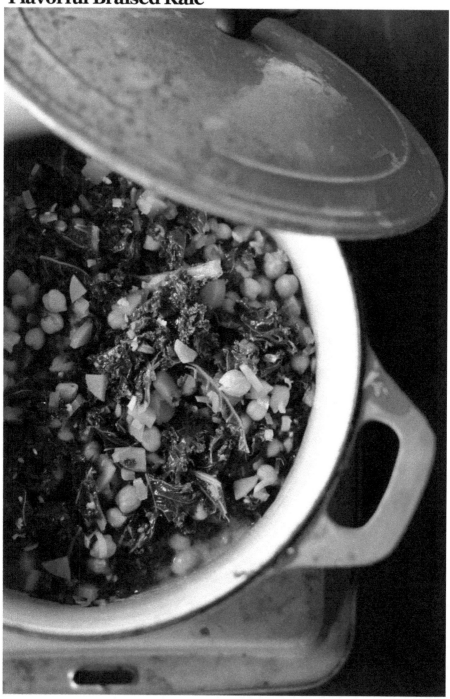

Difficulty Level: 2/5

Preparation time: 15 minutes

Cooking time: 15 minutes

Servings: 4

Ingredients:

1 lb. Kale, stems removed & chopped roughly

1 cup cherry tomatoes, halved

2 teaspoons olive oil

4 cloves garlic, sliced thin

½ cup vegetable stock

¼ teaspoon sea salt, fine

1 tablespoon lemon juice, fresh

1/8 teaspoon black pepper

Directions:

Start by heating your olive oil in a frying pan using medium heat, and add in your garlic. Sauté for a minute or two until lightly golden.

Mix your kale and vegetable stock with your garlic, adding it to your pan.

Cover the pan and then turn the heat down to medium-low.

Allow it to cook until your kale wilts and part of your vegetable stock should be dissolved. It should take roughly five minutes.

Stir in your tomatoes and cook without a lid until your kale is tender, and then remove it from heat.

Mix in your salt, pepper and lemon juice before serving warm.

Nutrition:
Calories: 70

Protein: 4 Grams

Fat: 0.5 Grams

Carbohydrates: 9 Grams

Sodium: 133 mg

Tomato and Wine-Steamed Mussels
Difficulty Level: 2/5

Preparation time: 10 minutes

Cooking time: 15 minutes

Servings: 4

Ingredients:

1 tablespoon olive oil

1 sweet onion, chopped

1 tablespoon minced garlic

1/8 teaspoon red pepper flakes

4 tomatoes, chopped

1/4 cup low-sodium fish or chicken stock

1/4 cup dry white wine

3 pounds mussels, cleaned and rinsed

Juice and zest of 1 lemon

1/4 cup pitted, sliced Kalamata olives

3 tablespoons chopped fresh parsley

Sea salt

Freshly ground black pepper

Directions:

In a large saucepan, heat the olive oil over medium-high heat. Sauté the onion, garlic, and red pepper flakes until softened, about 3 minutes. Stir in the tomatoes, stock, and wine and bring to a boil.

Add the mussels to the saucepan and cover. Steam until the mussels are opened, 6 to 7 minutes. Remove from the heat and discard any unopened shells.

Stir in the lemon juice, lemon zest, olives, and parsley. Season with salt and pepper and serve.

Nutrition:

Calories: 162

Total fat: 7g

Saturated fat: 1g

Carbohydrates: 12g

Sugar: 5g

Fiber: 3g

Protein: 12g

Citrus-Herb Scallops

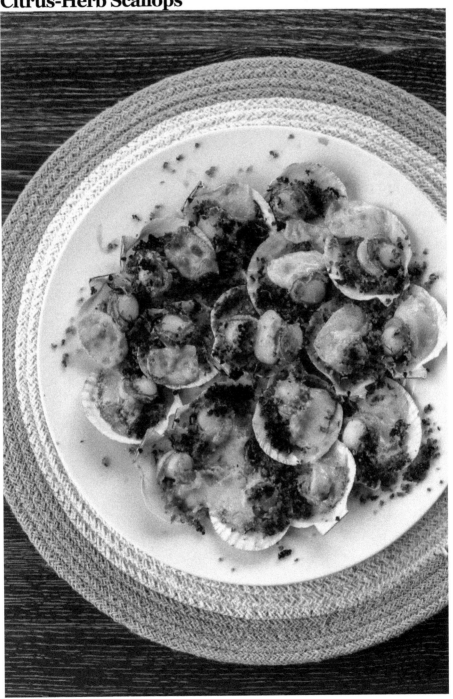

Difficulty Level: 2/5

Preparation time: 10 minutes

Cooking time: 4 minutes

Servings: 4

Ingredients:

1 pound sea scallops

Sea salt

Freshly ground black pepper

2 tablespoons olive oil

Juice of 1 lime

Pinch red pepper flakes

1 tablespoon chopped fresh cilantro

Directions:

Season the scallops lightly with salt and pepper.

In a large skillet, heat the olive oil over medium-high heat. Add the scallops to the skillet, making sure they do not touch one another.

Sear on both sides, turning once, for a total of about 3 minutes. Add the lime juice and red pepper flakes to the skillet and toss the scallops in the juice. Serve topped with cilantro.

Nutrition:

Calories: 160

Total fat: 8g

Saturated fat: 1g

Carbohydrates: 3g

Sugar: 0g

Fiber: 0g

Protein: 19g

Lightning Source UK Ltd.
Milton Keynes UK
UKHW020705310521
384670UK00006B/90